Diet Attitude

Change Your Attitude ~ Change Your Weight

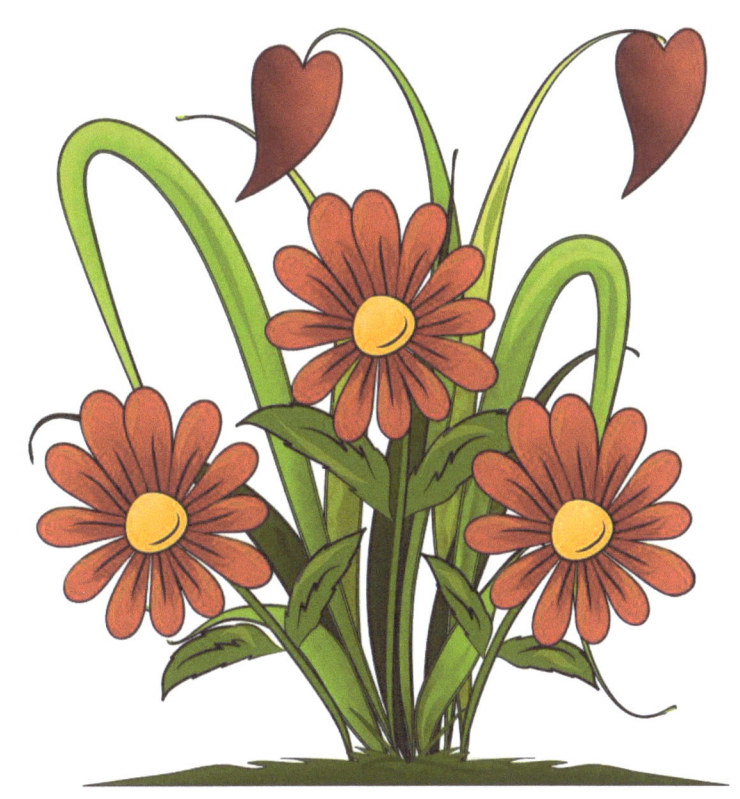

Written by Patricia Urato

BOGG Books
www.boggandco.com

Created using artwork by Trina Clark,
Alice Smith or Lisa Craig.

Scripture taken from the NEW AMERICAN STANDARD BIBLE®, Copyright ©
1960, 1962, 1963, 1968, 1971, 1972, 1973, 1975, 1977, 1995 by The Lockman Foundation.
Used by permission.

ISBN-13: 978-1475275568
ISBN-10: 1475275560

DEDICATION

This book is dedicated to all those
who have dieted.

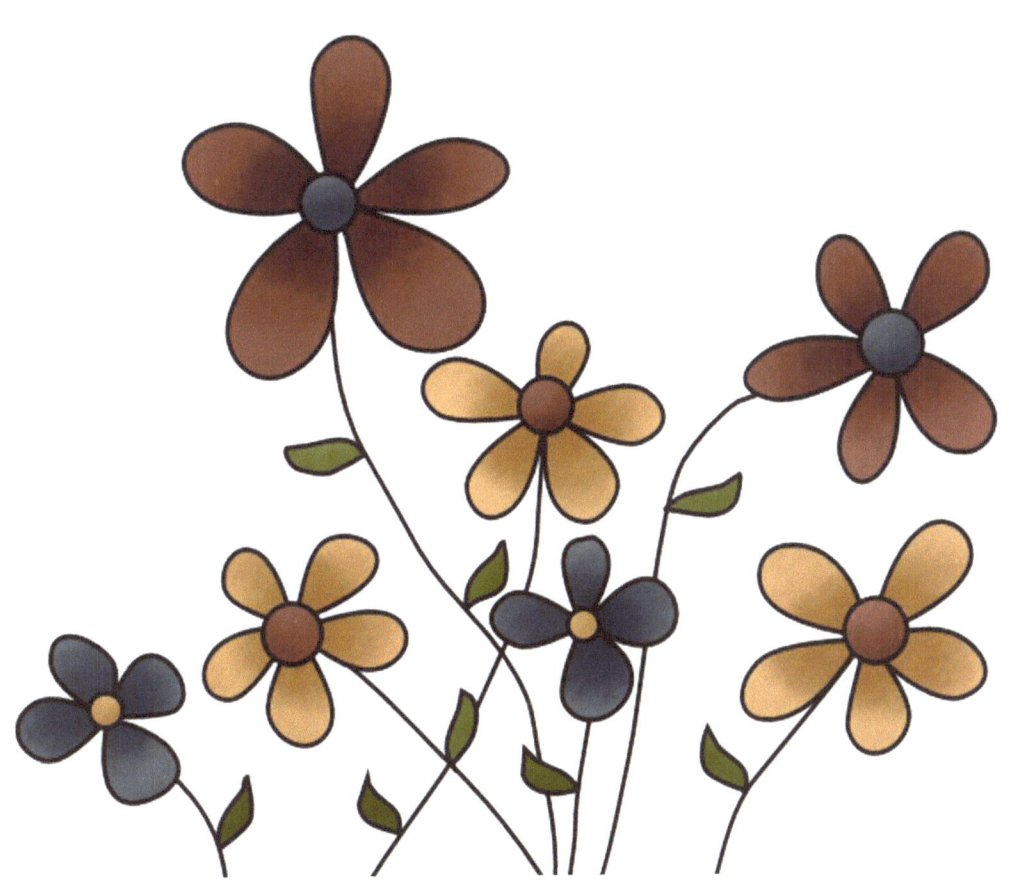

FORWARD

Dieting has never been easy and never will be. We are a society that celebrates everything with food and drink. We are a society that looks for comfort in food and drink.

Dieting isn't just about low carbs, low fat, calorie counting and exercise. Although all of these are important, dieting begins and ends with a positive attitude; a huge daily dose of positive attitude. Without it no diet will succeed.

It's alright to celebrate with food and drink but let's celebrate with control and with healthy food. And let's find an alternative for comfort.

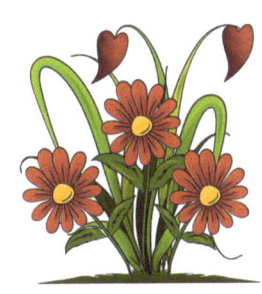

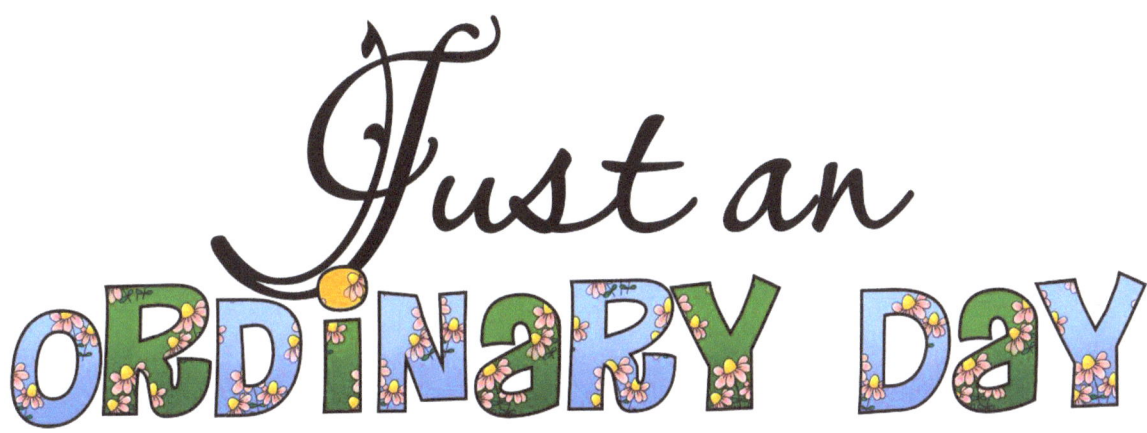

Just an ORDINARY DAY

Today is not just an ordinary day. Today is the day that you change your attitude and start eating healthy. Today is the day your attitude changes.

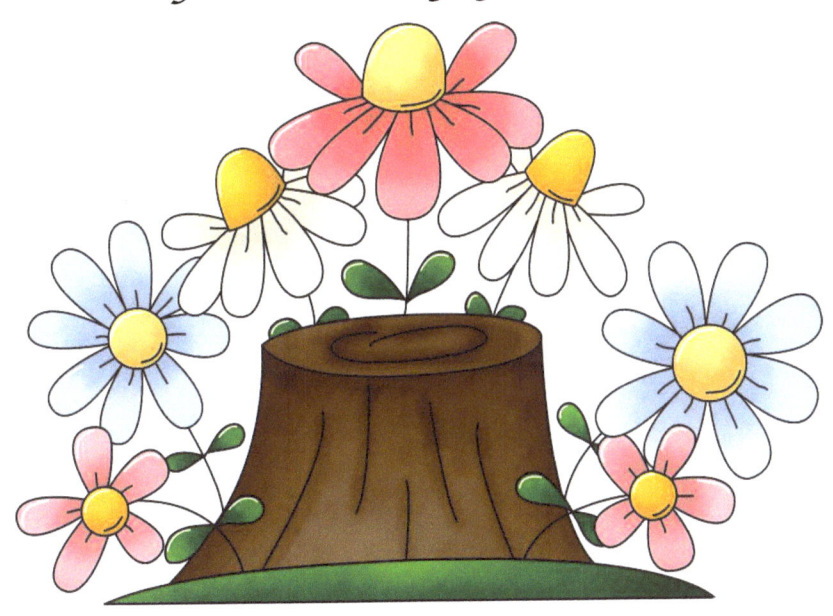

I am a BIG deal!

Acknowledge that you are important.

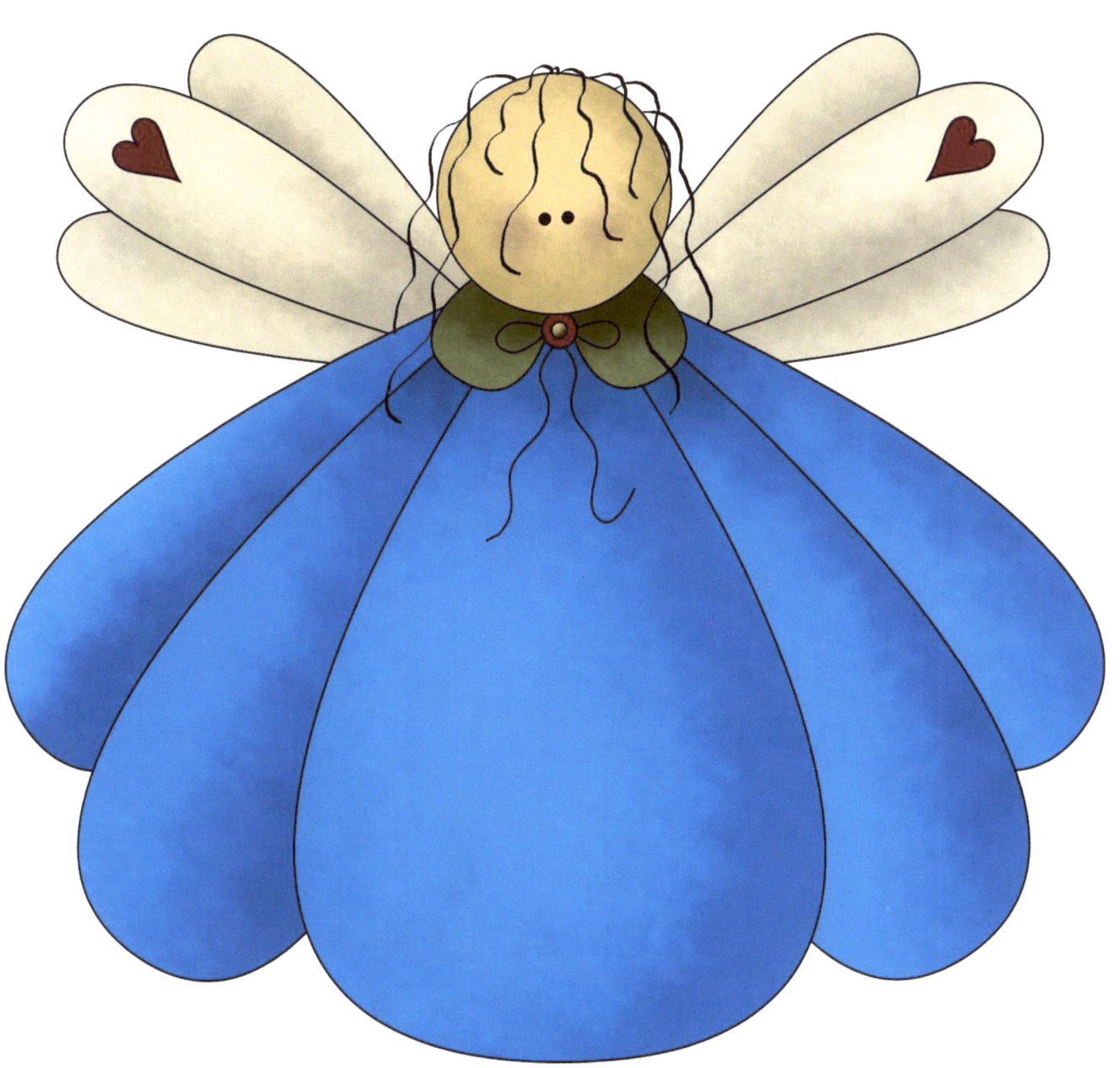

Slow and

steady

wins the

race.

~Aesop

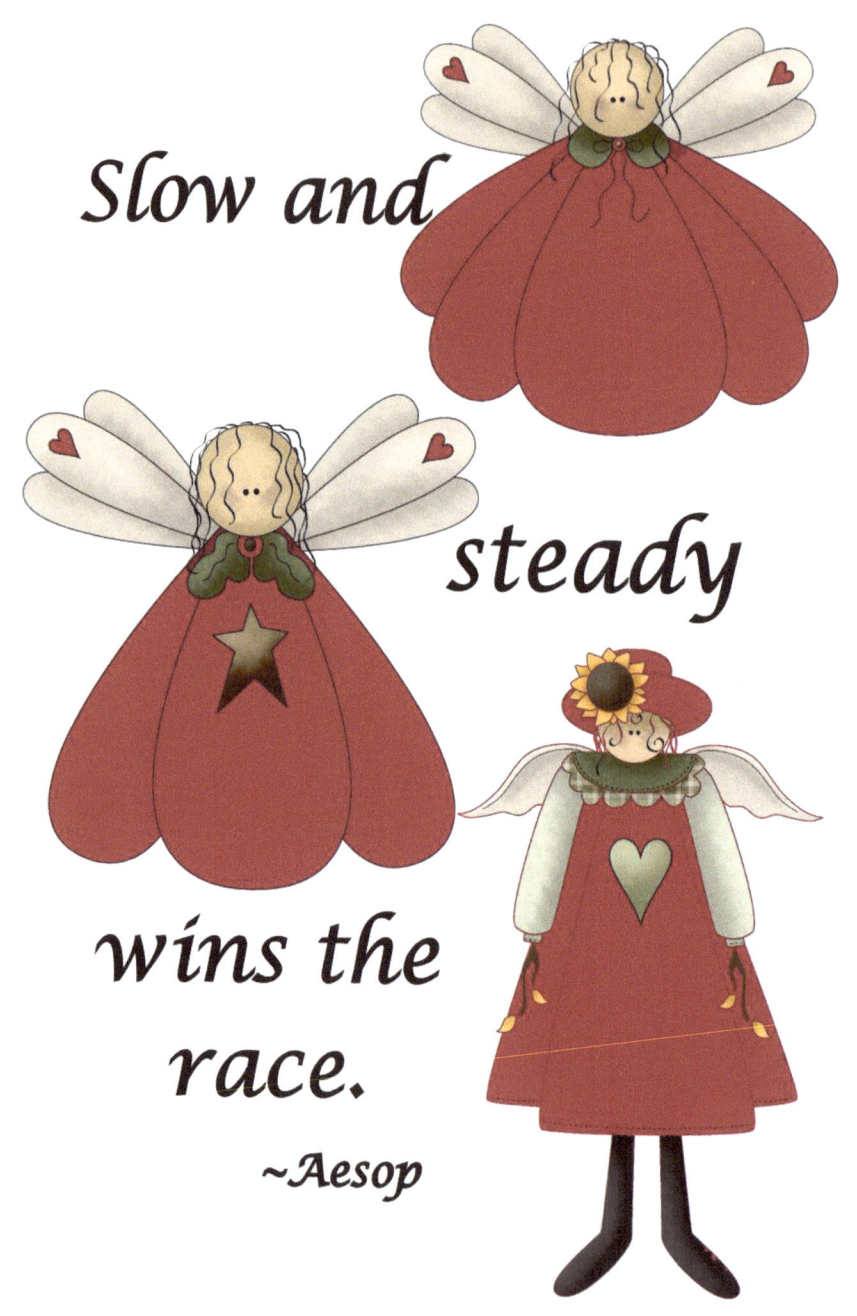

Subdue your appetites,
my dears, and you have
conquered human nature."

~ Charles Dickens

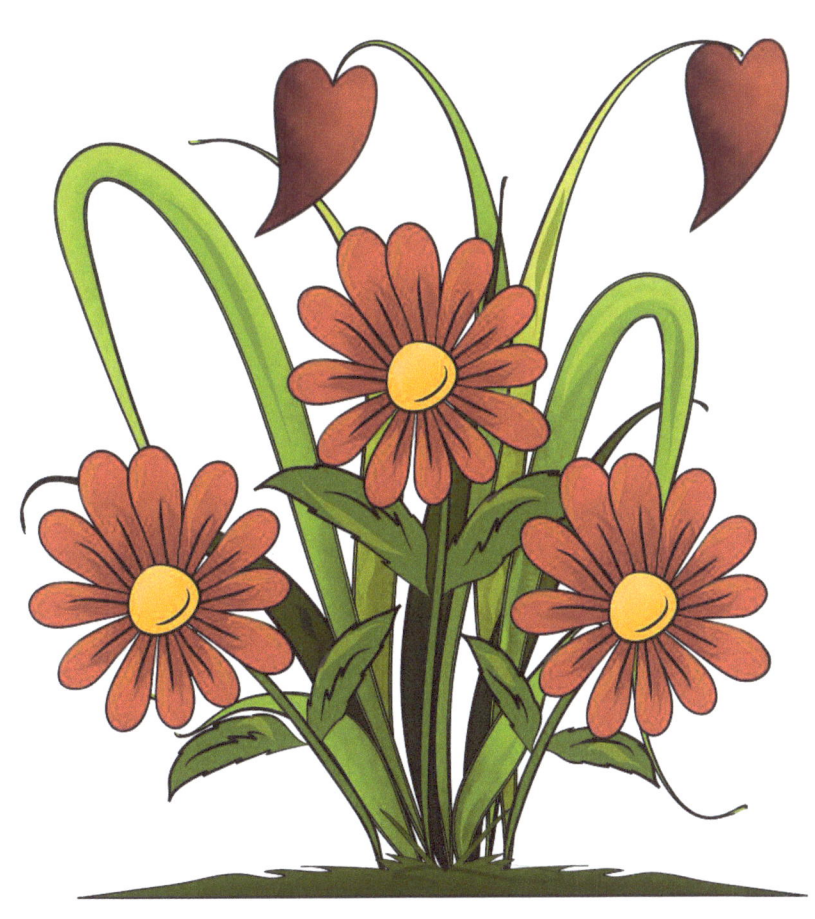

I keep trying to lose weight...
but it keeps finding me.

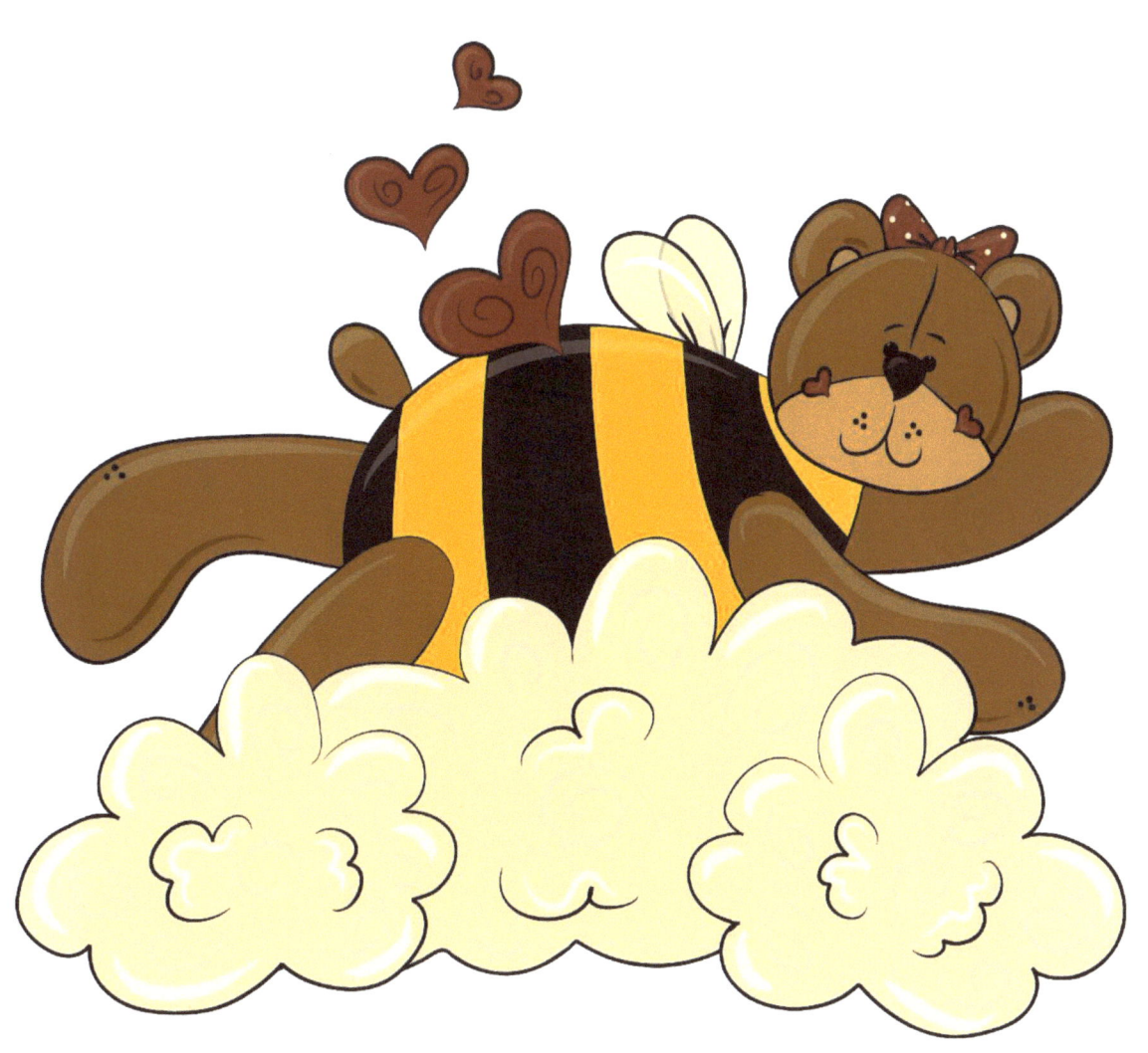

Blossom into the person you know you can be.

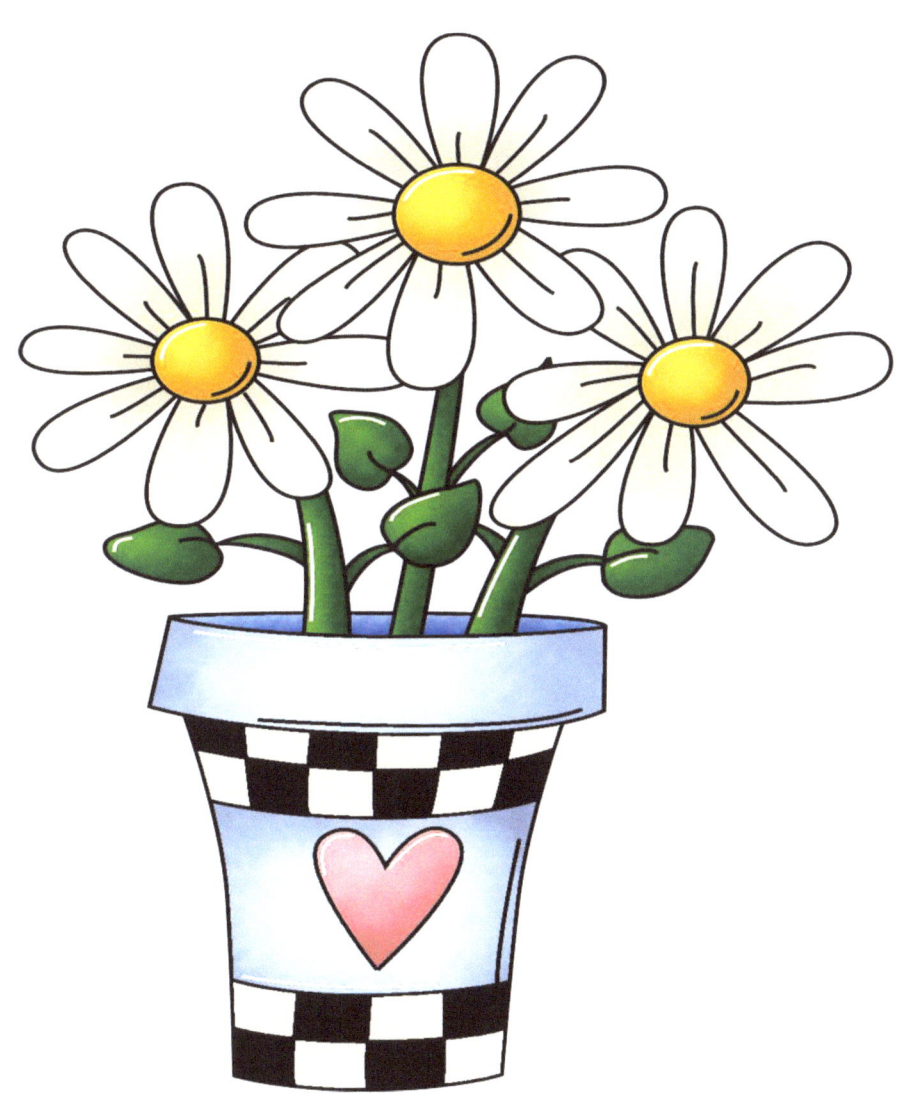

CAUTION!

Food Limit

When you exceed the food limit,
dieting is the penalty.

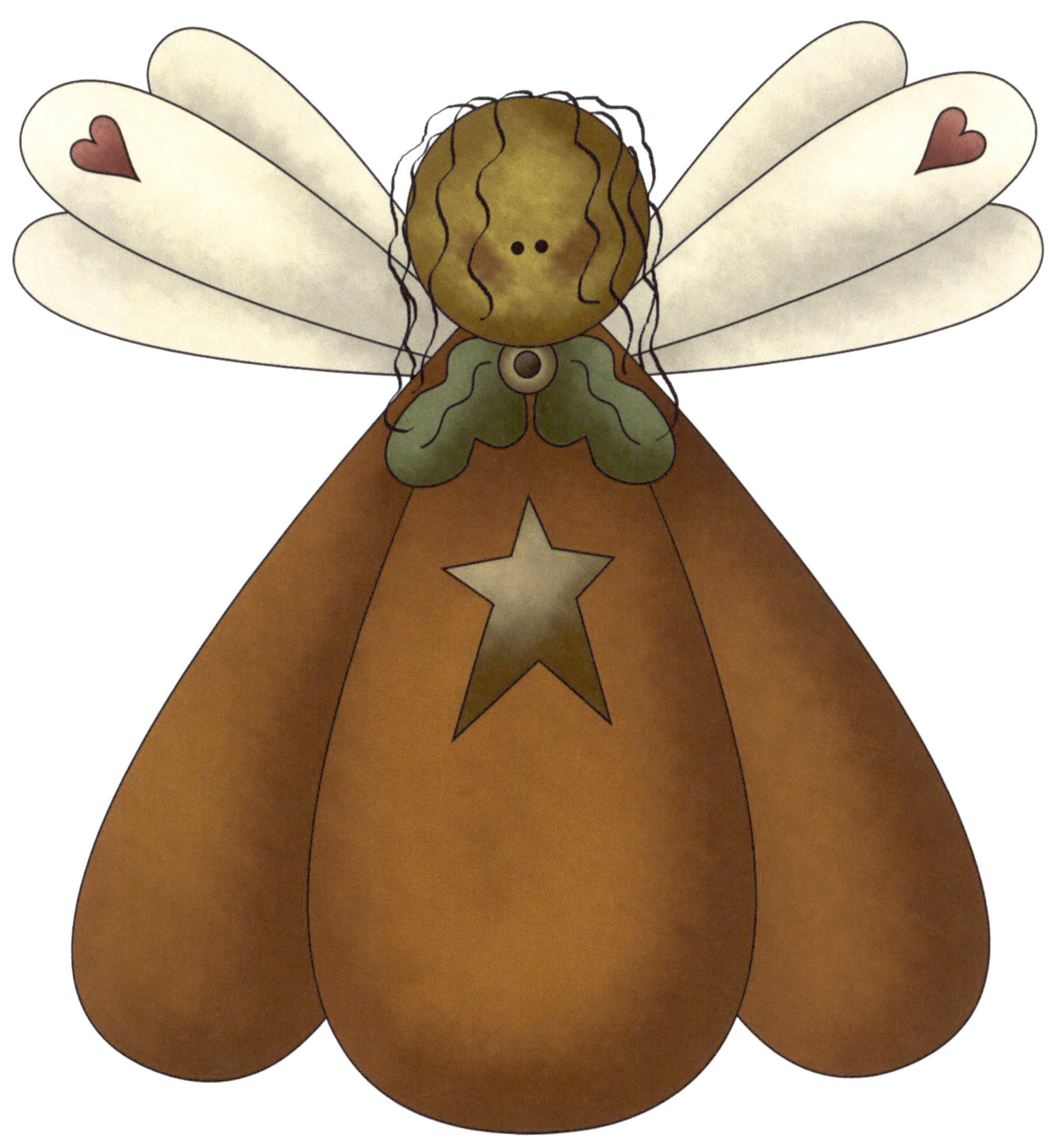

Give yourself
a shout out!

I am important!

I make a difference!

I am strong!

I can do all things through
Christ who strengthens me.

Happiness depends upon ourselves.

~Aristotle

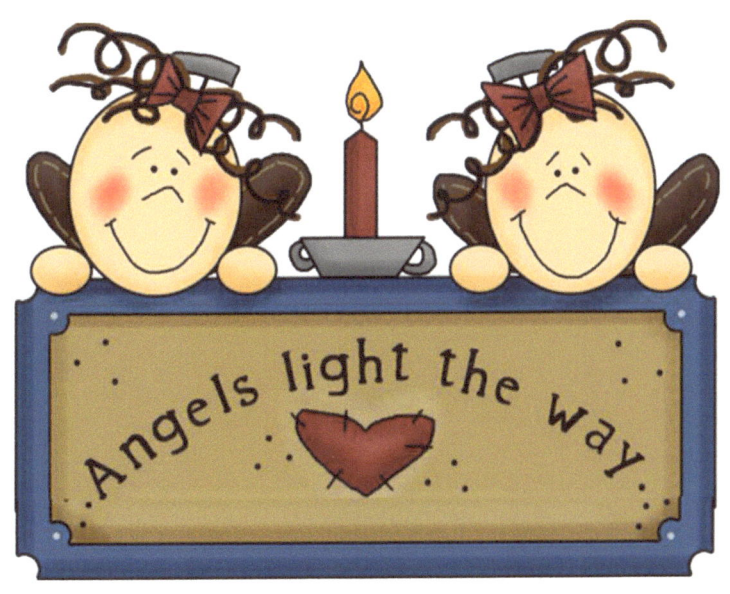

Are you overweight and unhappy?
Will you still be unhappy when you are thin?

Find your happiness first.

Both happiness and weight loss
begin with a positive attitude.

Love yourself.

Many of life's failures are people who did not realize how close they were to success when they gave up.

~ Thomas A. Edison

Don't set unrealistic expectations.
The weight went on slowly so it should
come off slowly.

Remember ~ Slow and steady wins the race.

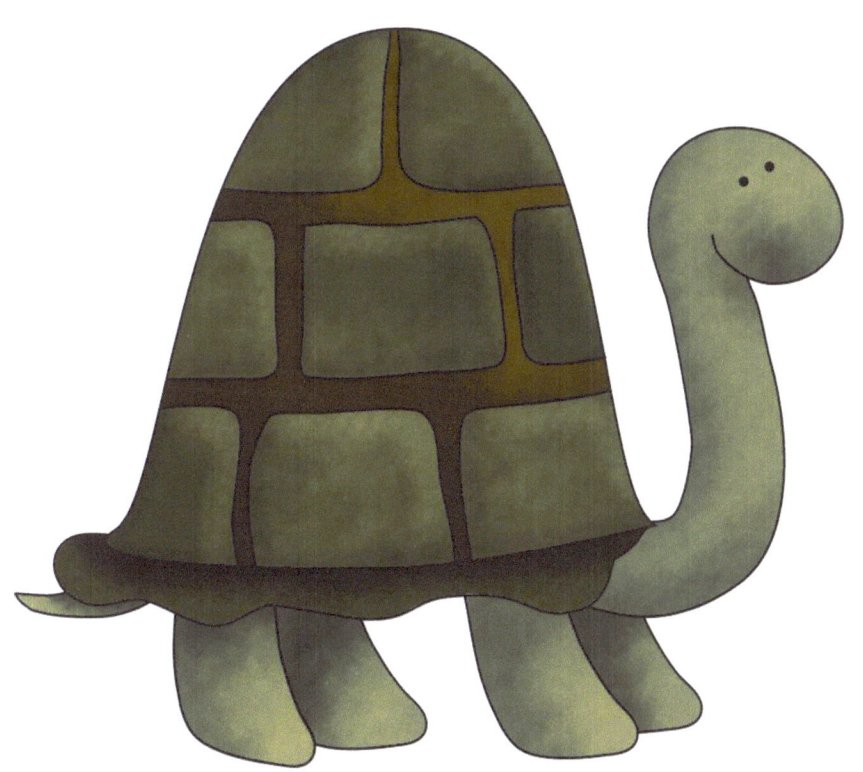

They can conquer who believe they can.

~ *Virgil*

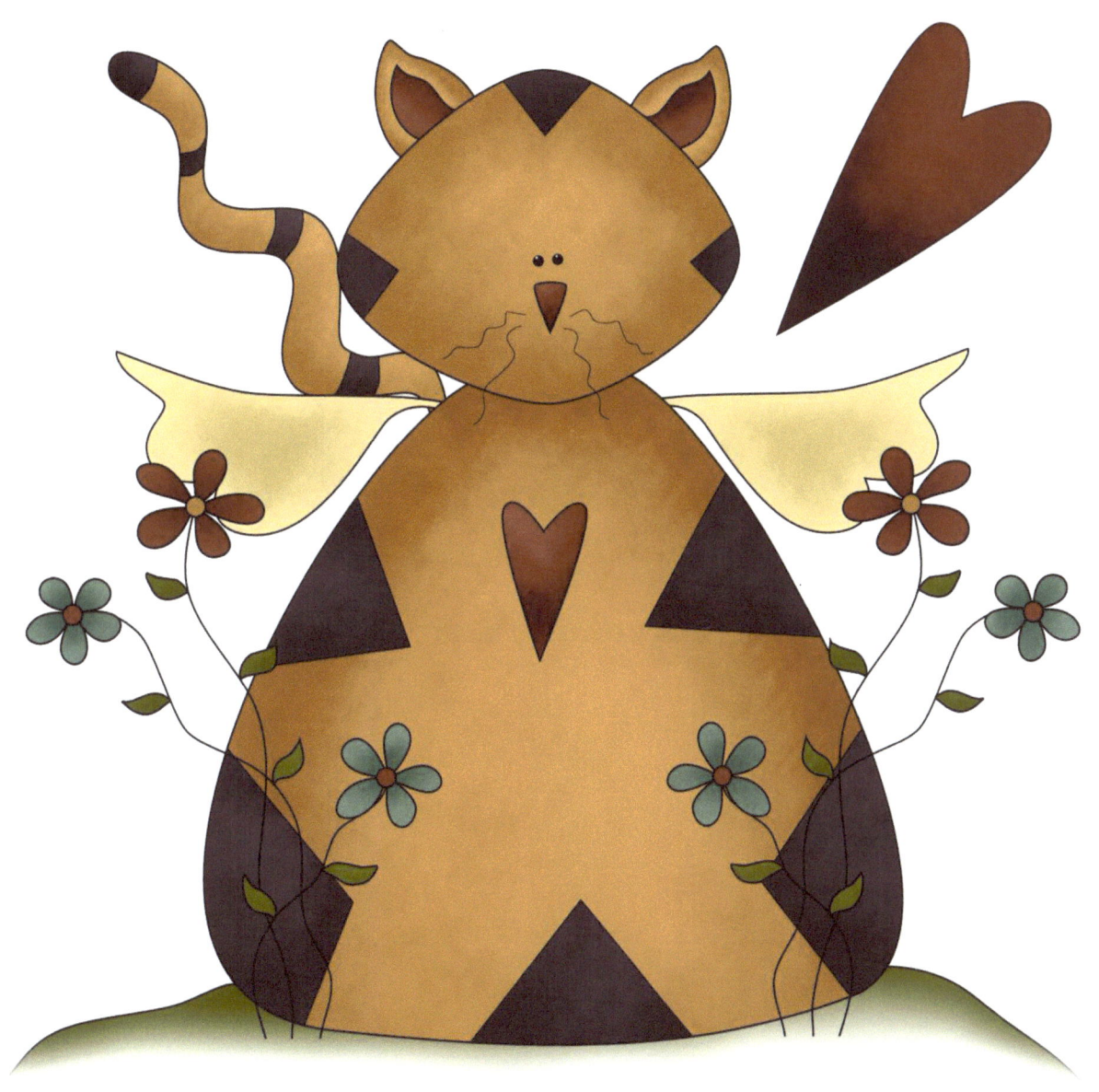

Believe

Blessed are those who hunger and thirst,
for they are sticking to their diets.

~ Author Unknown

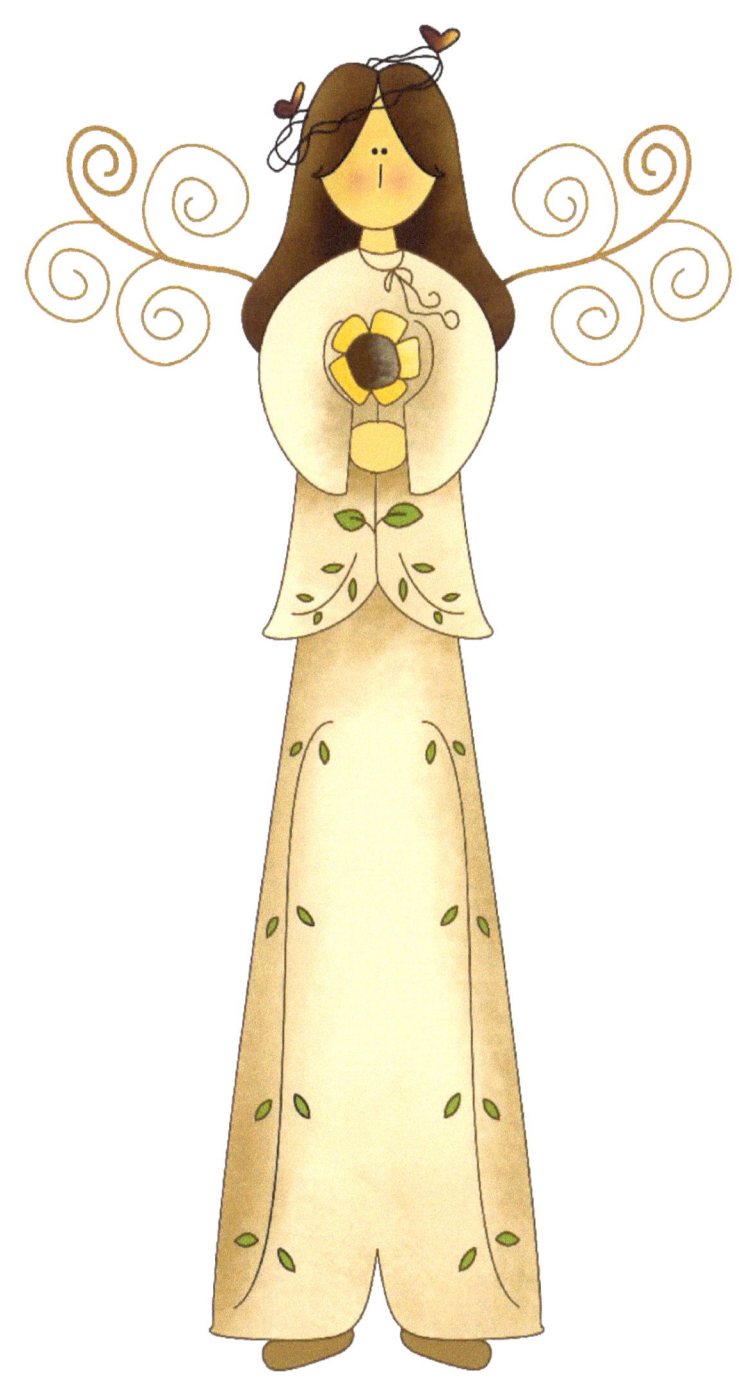

It's alright if you didn't stick with your diet today. Each day is a new beginning.

Finish each day and be done with it.
You have done what you can do.

~ Ralph Waldo Emerson

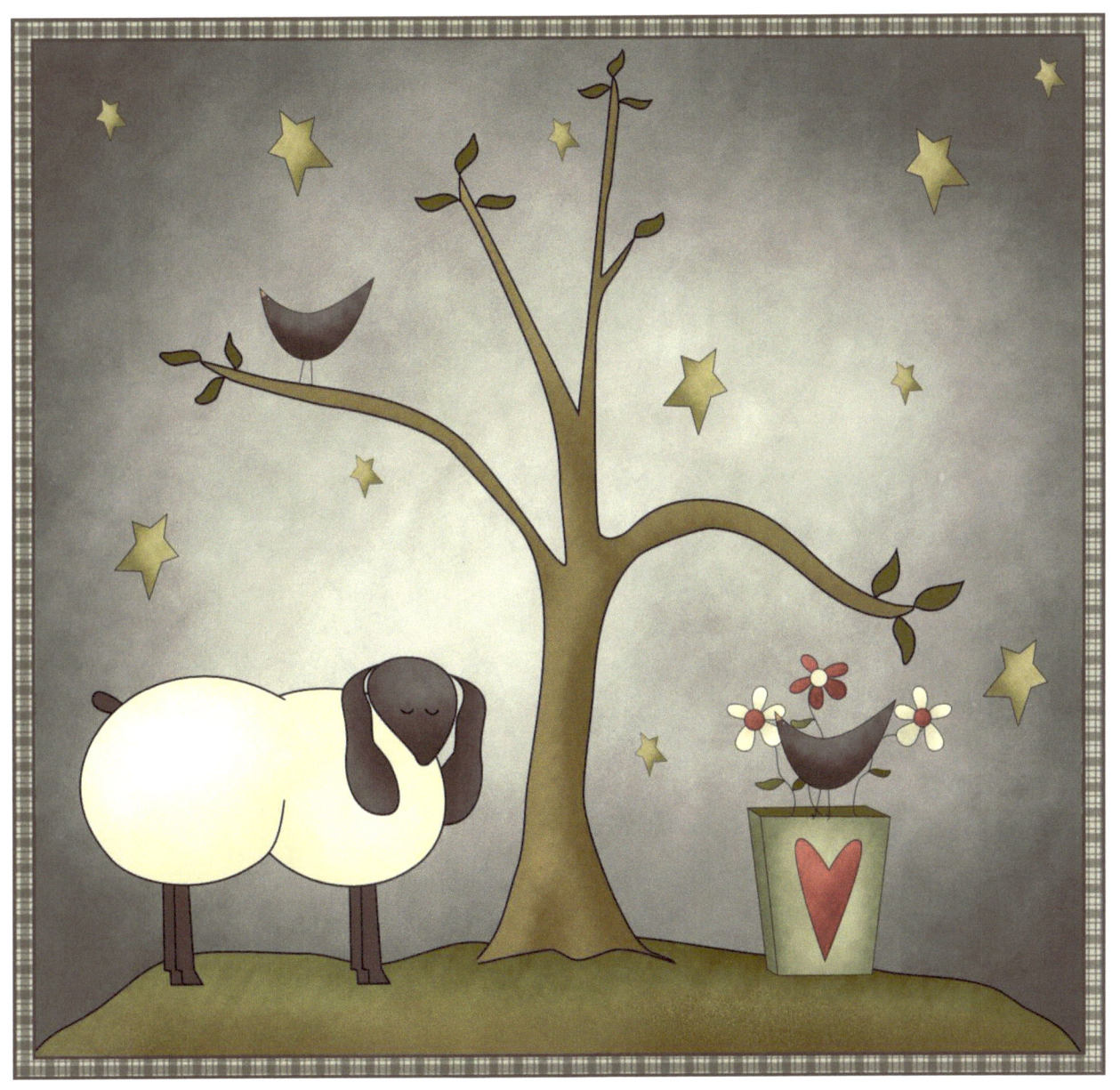

So do not worry about tomorrow; for tomorrow will care for itself.

~ Matthew 6:34

You didn't make me
a morning person, LORD.
But You did make
GREAT COFFEE.

Coffee Thyme

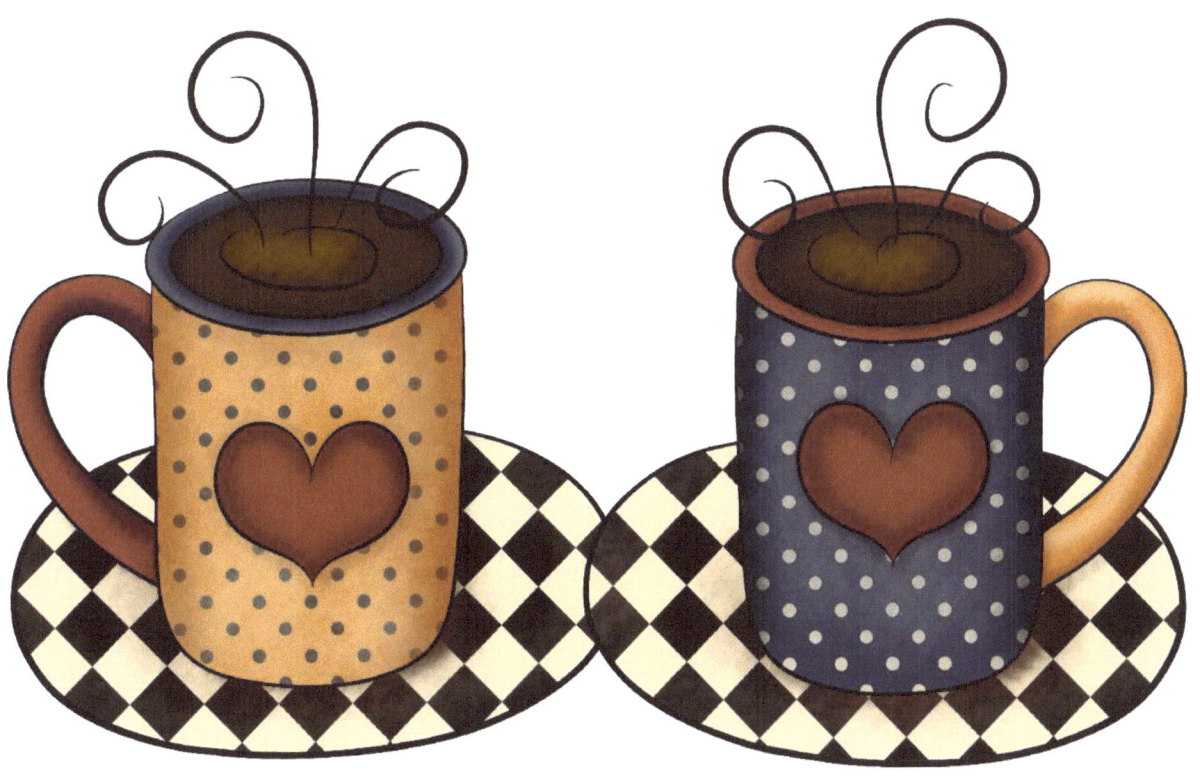

Dieting is not a piece of cake.

~Author Unknown

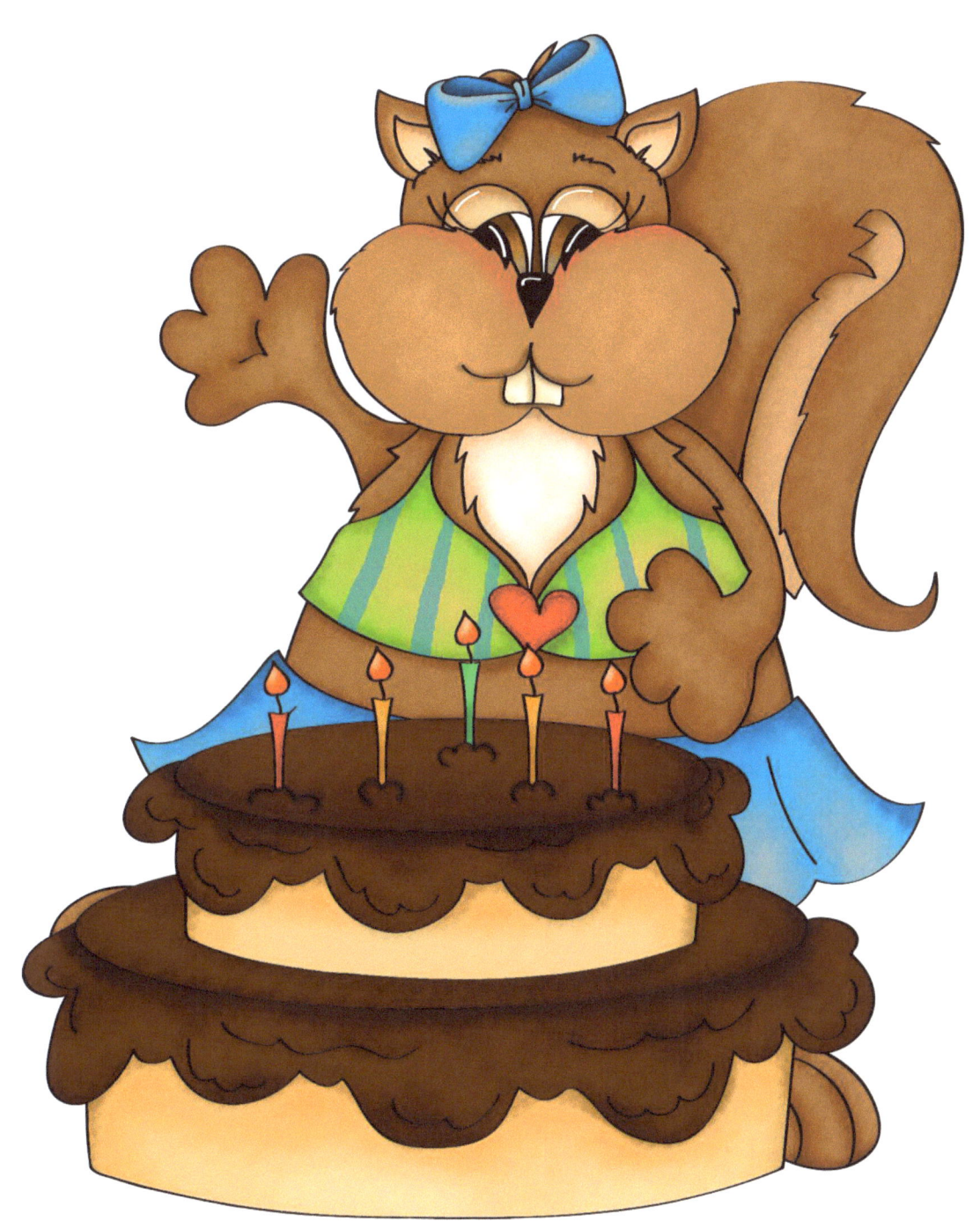

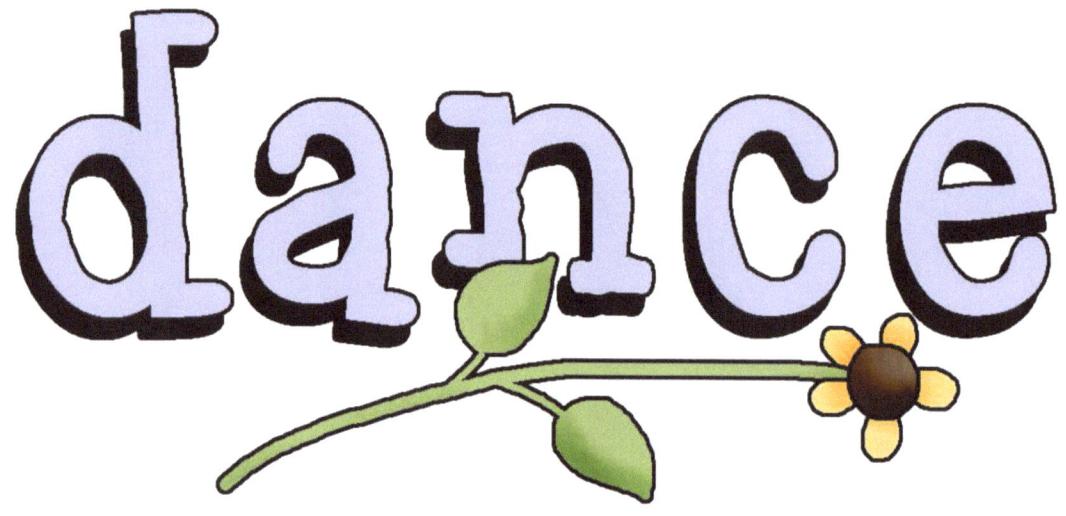

Dance the weight away!

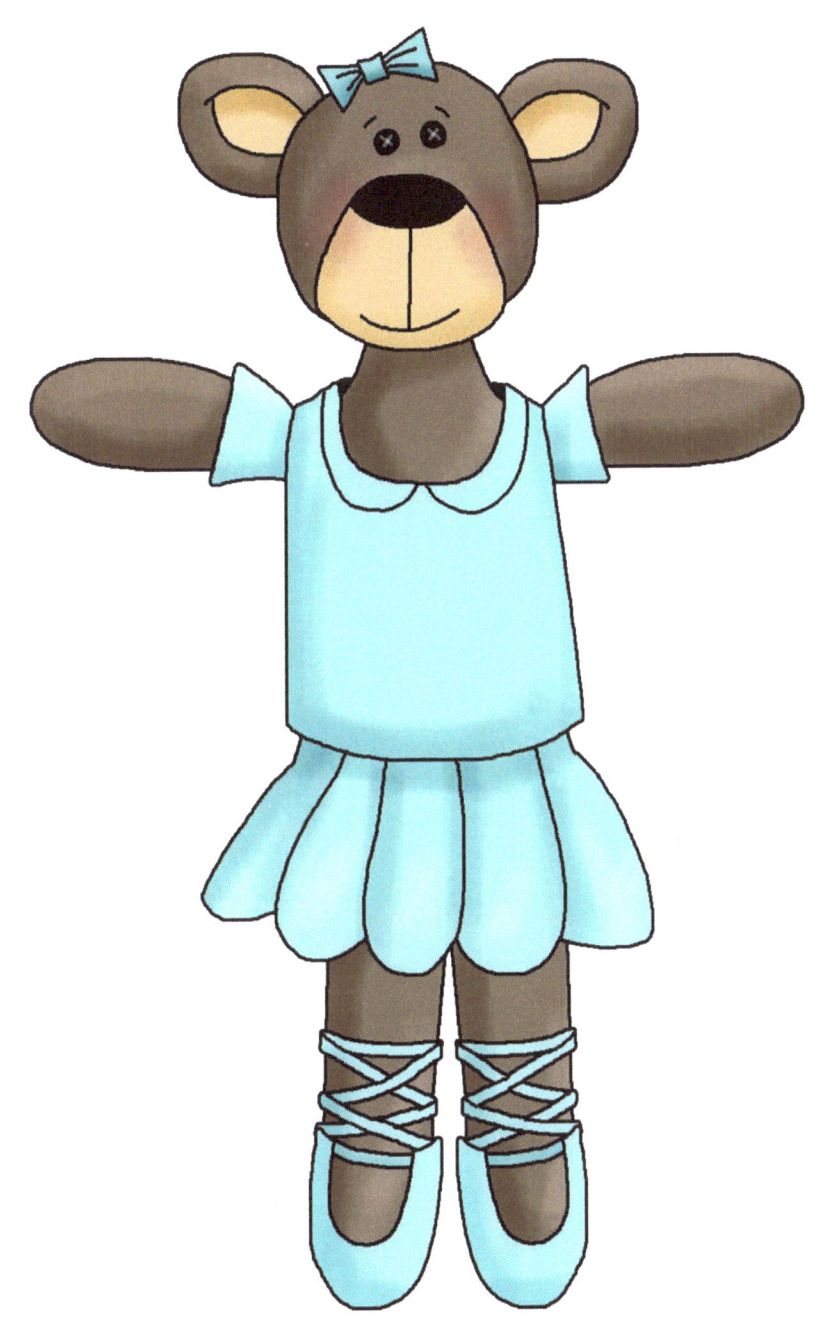

One should eat to live, not live to eat.

~Cicero

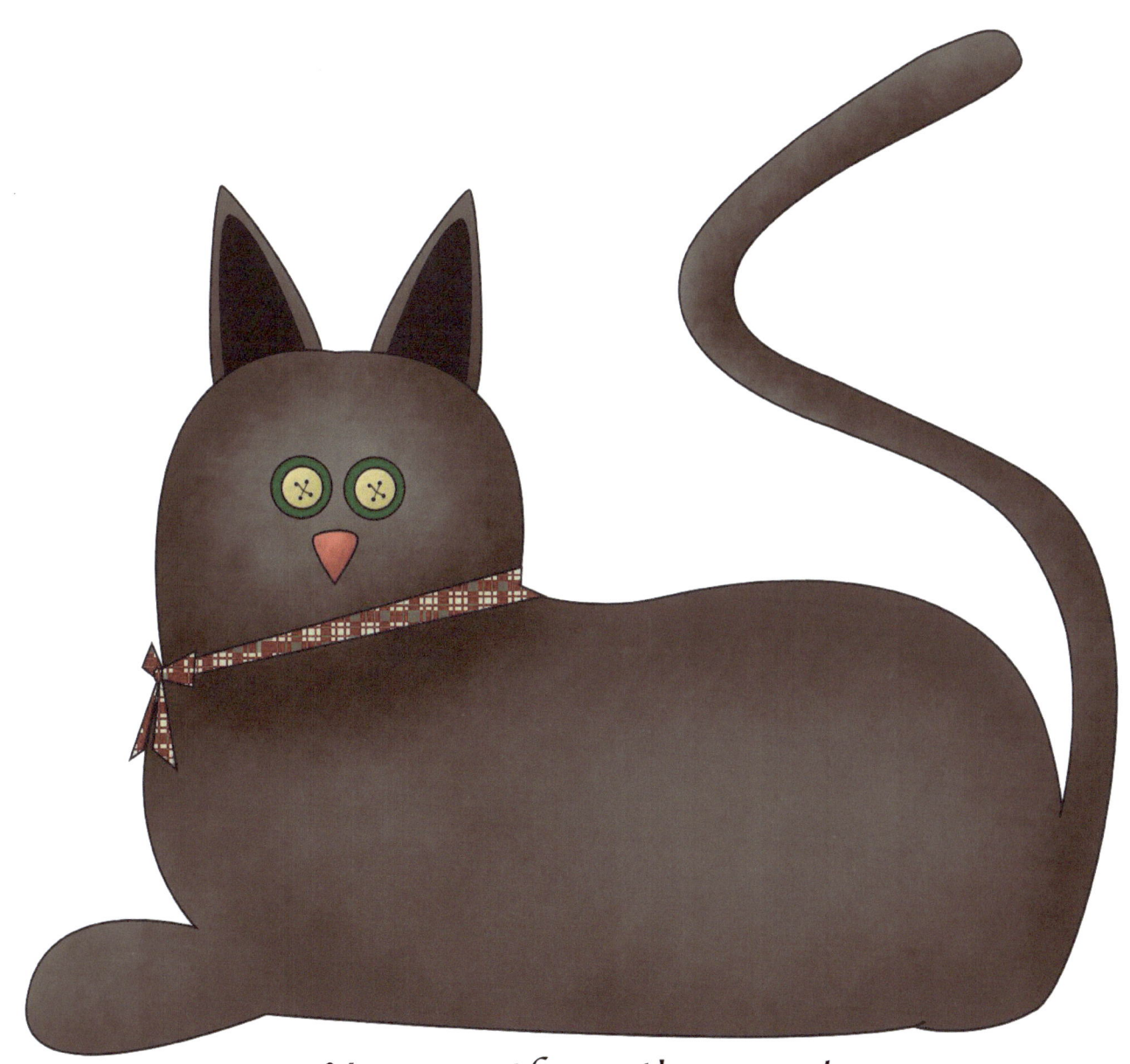

You are the cat's meow!

I have not failed. I've just found 10,000 ways that won't work.

~Thomas Edison

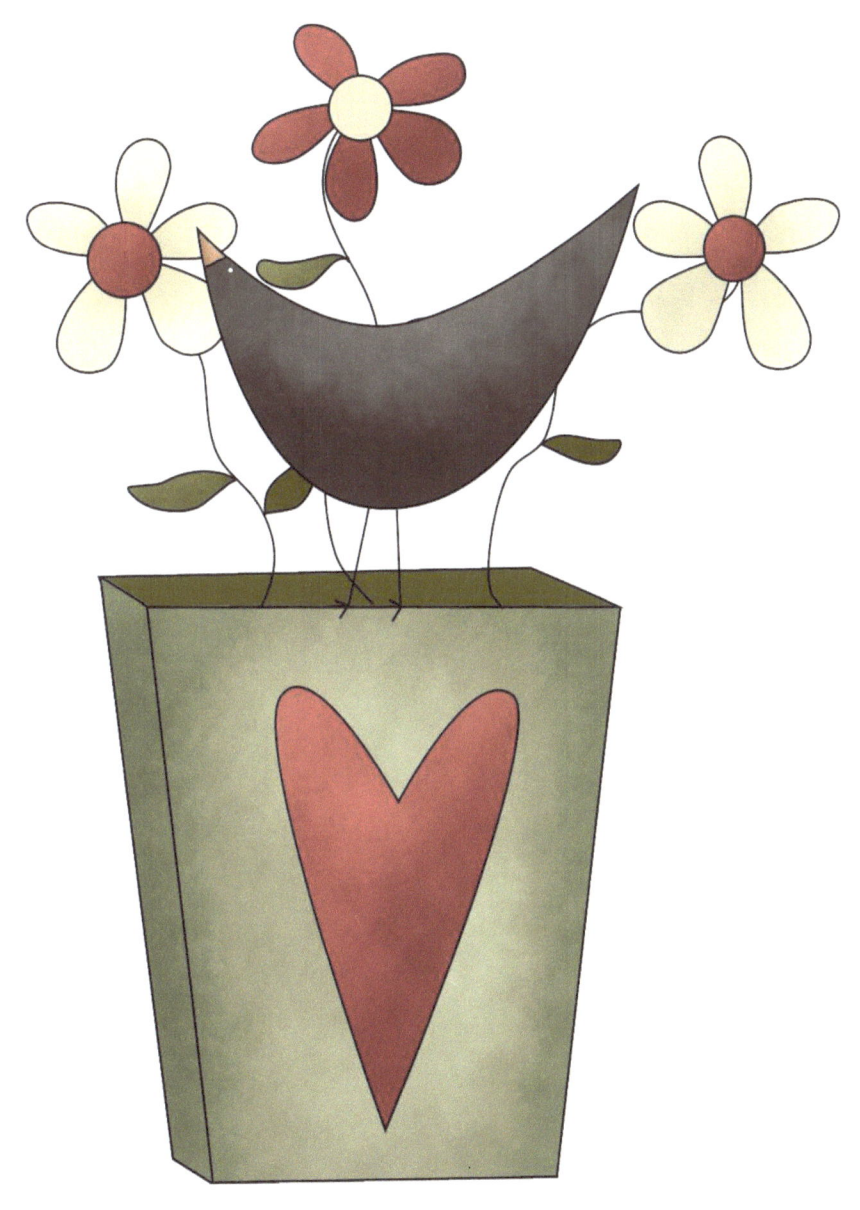

Find a diet that works for you.

When you are feeling stressed...

STOP...and watch the crocus pop through
the earth on a warm spring day.

STOP...and listen to the rhythm of the
ocean beating against the shore.

STOP...and enjoy the beauty of the
autumn foliage.

STOP...and listen to the silence of the
falling snow.

STOP...and feel the presence of God and listen
to Him as He guides you, comforts you
and instructs you in how to live a happy life.

~ Patricia Urato

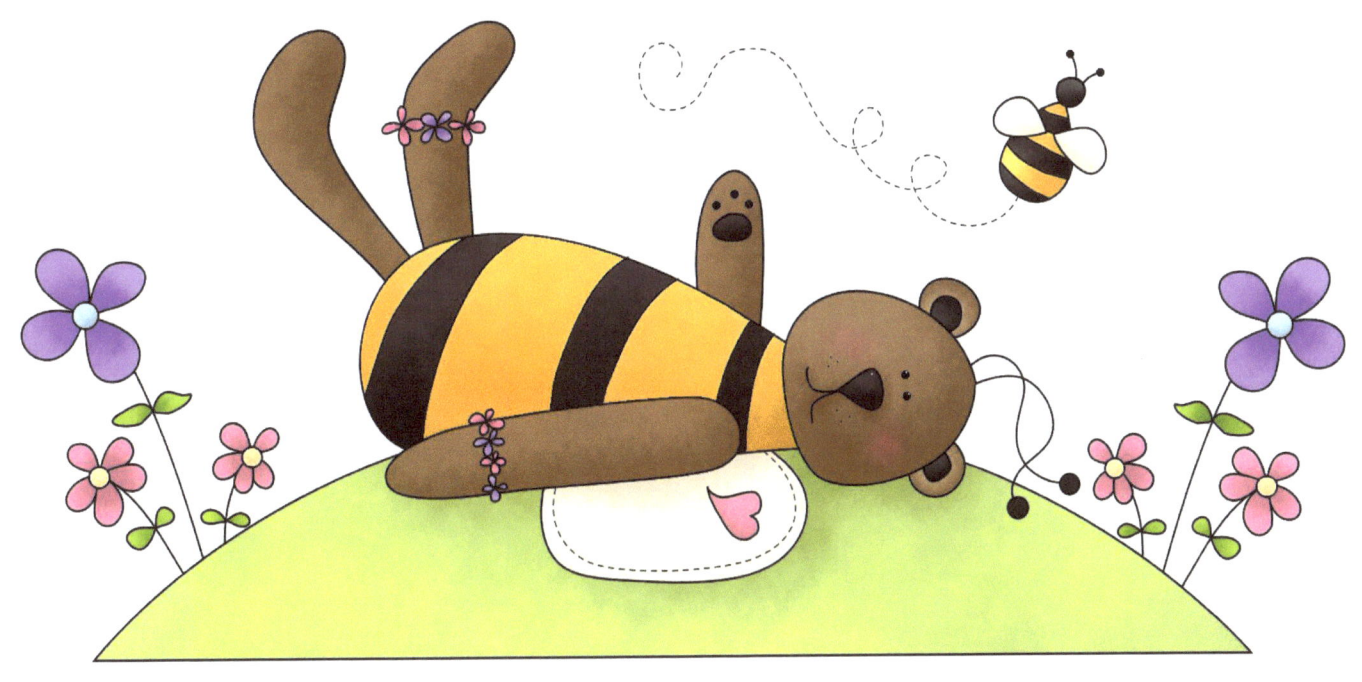

Take time to relax.

Journal
And Daily Affirmations

Journal
And Daily Affirmations

Journal

And Daily Affirmations

Journal

And Daily Affirmations

Journal
And Daily Affirmations

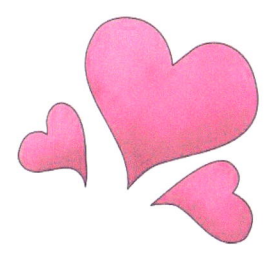

Journal

And Daily Affirmations

Journal

And Daily Affirmations

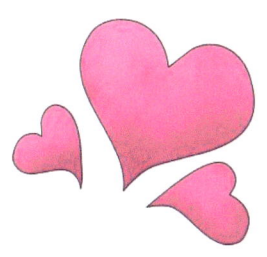

Journal

And Daily Affirmations

Journal
And Daily Affirmations

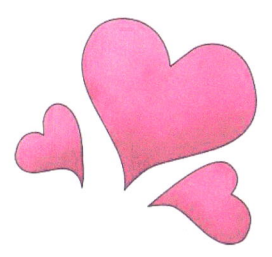

Journal
And Daily Affirmations

I tell you the truth, if you had faith even as small as a mustard seed, you could say to this mountain, 'Move from here to there,' and it would move. Nothing would be impossible.

~ Matthew 17:20